Chinese Health Balls

Other books by Binkey Kok Publications

Eva Rudy Jansen
Singing Bowls
A Practical Handbook of Instruction and Use

The Book of Buddhas
Ritual Symbolism Used
on Buddhist Statuary and Ritual Objects

Eva Rudy Jansen
The Book of Hindu Imagery
The Gods and their Symbols

Hans Höting

Chinese Health Balls

Practical Exercises

Binkey Kok Publications, Diever, Holland

CIP-DATA KONINKLIJKE BIBLIOTHEEK, DEN HAAG

Höting, Hans

Chinese health balls : practical exercises / Hans Höting ;
[transl. from the German by Tony Langam ... et al. ;
photo's Bert Wieringa ; ill. Franz Kossek]. − Diever ;
Binkey Kok. − Ill., photo's
Transl. of: Aktiv und gesund durch die magischen
Gigong-Kugeln aus China. − Bremen : Höting, 1989. − With index.
ISBN 90-74597-03-3
Subject headings: Chinese health balls / alternative medicine.

Published and © by Binkey Kok Publications
Diever Holland. Fax 31 5219 1925.

Printed and bound in the Netherlands.
Lay-out: Eva Rudy Jansen
Cover design: Jaap Koning.

Distributed in the U.S.A. by
Samuel Weiser Inc., Box 612, York Beach, Maine 03910.

Contents

Foreword

Increasingly, Asian ideas, customs and objects are finding their way into our shops and homes. We simply like many of these objects, or consider them beautiful or useful - at least, if we are interested in them. But some of them give rise to questions. What is it ? What's it for ? What do you do with it ?

This category of intriguing objects includes the oblong boxes lined with colourful embroidered silk, containing two balls, usually made of metal. The balls feel heavy in the hand, and when you move them, they make a bell-like sound. They are sold under various different names, and usually all that is said is that you should roll them around in your hand. In most cases it remains a mystery what this rolling is good for, or what else you could do with the balls.

We have already made two successful attempts at unveiling these "Eastern mysteries": first in a book about the use and effects of singing bowls, and then in a concise iconography of Tibetan Buddhism. For this third publication in our series, we were able to use a German book, which not only provides accurate information about the background and effect of the mysterious metal balls, but also contains an extensive series of exercises, so that the reader can start investigating the effect of the balls for himself straightaway. For our English and American readers, we have produced a modified version of this book, which we hope is comprehensive; we have tried to adapt the content as far as possible to their wishes and interests.

The publisher

Introduction

One of the ways in which man is distinct from all other living crea-
tures is the fact that he has never been able to accept the natural
cycle of birth, sickness and death. From the time that man first walked the earth, he has been looking for ways of preventing illness and
extending life. There are countless sagas, fairytales and folk tales
about the sources of eternal youth, elixirs of life, magical herbs and
other miracle cures. Many of these stories can be lumped together as
the well-known phenomenon of "wishful thinking", but many contain a kernel of truth. The truth is that popular medicine has always
made use of methods which activate the excretory functions,
strengthen natural resistance, and stimulate the circulation of the
blood. These three basic principles of natural medicine are used
throughout the world, because they do actually promote health, and
therefore, under certain circumstances, even prolong life.
The ways in which these three principles operate are apparently
often very different. However, a critical examination shows that
there is always one great similarity, because whichever method is
used, it is never more than a remedy, an initial impetus. The most
important factor in healing is man himself. Without him making an
effort, even the best medicine in the world has little chance of
succeeding.

The view that physical health goes hand in hand with mental and
emotional health is generally accepted nowadays. A person's ap-
proach to life influences how he feels. The best known example of

this is possibly that of ulcers caused by repressed tension.

Health is a matter of balance in mind, emotions and body. Any disturbance in this balance, particularly if it is a long-term disturbance, can result in illness. In this case the healing process consists of restoring the balance. Sometimes this is a short route, but if the disturbance has lasted a long time, the path back is also a matter of time, and therefore, above all, of perseverance. No medicine can work if it is not given the time to work.

If there is one method for which this applies, it must be that of Chinese health balls. They can provide a healing therapy which is closely related to acupuncture and reflexology. They have the advantage that a person can use them himself without any outside help. But anyone who expects to be fit and healthy after using these balls for a short time, will be sorely disappointed. The positive effect of Chinese health balls, the subject of this book, only really comes into its own after long-term use. Thus they certainly do not act as a "miracle cure", but they are a very pleasant method of healing, a wonderful activity, and this activity in itself has a certain therapeutic value because it has a relaxing effect on the body as well as the mind.

This book describes in detail the demonstrable effect, which is based on the principles of the medicine of the Far East, as well as the fascinating background of the balls. It also contains a large number of applications in the form of practical exercises.

May your journey be an agreeable one.

Part 1

Origins

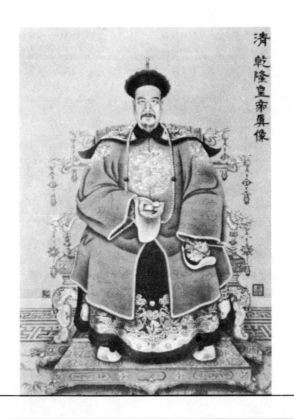

清 乾隆皇帝真像

History

Anyone who has had the opportunity to travel around China will undoubtedly have come across people there who are simply standing or sitting around, apparently lost in thought... The only movement you see is that of two or three balls being rotated in the palm of their hand. At first sight, this seems a way of passing the time which has no deeper meaning, an unconscious game, just as we might play with an elastic band or a few paperclips. But this is very deceptive. In reality, we are concerned here with an ancient Chinese fitness technique.

The balls which are now made in China, and which also find their way to our country, are made in the Baoding factory, amongst other places. This factory's archives reveal that during the Han Dynasty (206 BC − 230 AD), walnuts were used for hand training, while manuscripts from the Sung Dynasty (960 − 1280 AD) show that the use of real balls was already established for this purpose. Initially they were used particularly in the martial arts as weapons, and by acrobats as props to demonstrate their skills. It was only during the Ming Dynasty (1368-1644) that the balls were used on a large scale for their positive effect on health. The Emperor Cha Ching from this dynasty introduced them at his court after he had seen a large number of his vassals using them, and had instigated an inquiry into their effect. In fact, the Ming Dynasty was an important period in the history of Chinese health balls, because until that time, solid balls had been used. It was only in the Ming Dynasty that a process was developed for the manufacture of hollow balls.

The Emperor Kwan Long in the Ching Dynasty, who reigned from 1736-1796, was advised by his physician to exercise with the balls every day. This emperor was so enthusiastic that he developed a cult based on them, and had all sorts of special objects d'art made. He lived to the age of eighty-nine, his physician to the age of eighty-four. The famous Chinese painter, Qi Baishe, also used the health balls and lived to be ninety-eight !

Today, a large number of prominent Chinese figures − artists and sportsmen − still use the balls to stay fit and promote their physical and mental health.

The Principle

To understand the principle on which the effect of Chinese health balls is based, it is useful to know more about Chinese philosophy and the healing methods derived from it. According to this Chinese philosophy, not only life on earth, but ultimately the existence of the whole universe, is based on the principle of duality. The beginning is complemented by the end, dark produces light, day is a product of night. White exists only because black exists, sound can be heard because it issues forth from silence. We experience joy because there is sorrow. The blossoming of spring and the full life of summer are followed by the dying autumn and the apparent death of winter. Everything consists of two opposing poles. In Chinese philosophy these two polarities are described by the terms **yin** and **yang**, which have gradually become familiar in the West as well. Yin represents the female principle, the wet, dark, passive side; yang represents the male principle, the dry, light, active side. When yin and yang are in balance, there is harmony and health.

Each is dependent on the other, without one the other cannot exist, and in addition, when one increases, the other decreases. The energy produced by the eternal polarity between yin and yang is called **ki** (also written: qi or chi).

Ki is life energy, the force which moves, controls and regulates everything. Without ki there is no life, and conversely, without life there is no ki. It should be remembered that ki is not only a philosophical principle, it is a unit which exists in concrete form, a specific form of energy.

After all, we do not say that matter is merely a philosophical principle, simply because it is a particular form of energy. And yet, it is
actually no more than that, or, as Albert Einstein said: 'Energy has
mass, and mass represents energy.' A Buddhist sutra formulates
this concept in the following words: 'Form is emptiness and emptiness is form. Emptiness is not distinct from form, and form is not distinct from emptiness.' The physicist and author, Fritjof Capra, who
became famous for his book, *The Tao of Physics*, described the idea in
the following words: 'Through the discovery that particles are
created spontaneously in a void, and then disappear in a void, we
have permanently had to abandon the distinction between matter
and empty space.'

Insights such as these, in which Eastern philosophy and Western
science come together, completely accept the existence of a driving
force which controls the creation and disappearance of all forms of
matter. It is this force which is given the name **ki**.

According to the Chinese view, ki is present in the universe as primal ki, the force from which everything was created originally, and
from which everything is constantly being created, the primal force
which directs and controls the universe.

Ki is present in the body in various different forms, each with its own
function. For example, there is the ki in the organs, the force which
enables the organs to function, the ki in the respiration, the force
which enters the body when we breathe, and the ki of digestion,
which we take in with our food, and which replenishes our reserve of
energy when we have used some of it up in physical activity or illness. Our parents passed ki on to us at conception and birth. Ki circu-
lates throughout our entire body through the acupuncture meridians. Acupuncture makes use of this system by means of needles
which are placed in these channels of energy at special points.

However, there are many other techniques which are aimed at restoring, activating and stimulating the passage of ki in the body. According to the Chinese healing methods, tried and tested for centuries,
and which are based on the ki principle, illnesses can be traced back
to disturbances in the passage of ki. There are various different techniques aimed at restoring the balance of ki. A number of these have
become well known in the west, and have even been adopted on a
large scale. In the first place, there is the above-mentioned method
of acupuncture, but in addition, Tai-Chi (a movement technique),

Rei Ki (a technique in which the passages of ki are activated by means of the direct transmission of energy, and Qi-Gong (a breathing technique) are becoming increasingly well known. Ki techniques have a quantifiable influence on the cerebral cortex, the autonomic nervous system, the circulation of the blood, and digestion.

Chinese health balls also affect the passage of ki along the channels of energy in our body. In Chinese hospitals they have been used for this purpose for many years.

Terminology

The balls which are available in various different types − this is
described in detail later on − are known by different names. Sometimes they are called Baoding balls; this name is taken from one of
the most important factories in China which manufactures them.
Another name is Qi-Gong balls, after the technique of the same
name. 'Gong' is a Chinese word for 'working'; therefore Qi-Gong
means 'working on the energy'.
In China itself, there are at least two common names: 'Baichi', which
means 'valuable balls', and 'Baodjan Chu', which means 'health
balls'.
As for our own language: the term 'chiming balls' is used sometimes,
relating to the sound that some, though not all, types of balls produce.
Because of all these different names, it seemed best not to confuse
matters even further, but simply use the straightforward, appropriate name, 'Chinese health balls', in this book.

Part 2

The Effects

As Chinese health balls have been used in China for such a long time, also in hospitals, there is extensive written documentation on the results of the practice. These medical reports reveal that patients have experienced remarkable improvements for all sorts of complaints by working intensively with the balls for a long period of time. One might be inclined to dismiss these stories as yet another series of funny medical miracle fables, if there were not a number of explanations for the real influence which the use of the balls has on the human organism. In this chapter, we will briefly outline a number of these explanations. If you would like to study this in more detail, you should read other books about the various methods of examination and healing dealt with below. In this book we can only provide a general description, in so far as there is a relationship or correspondence between the technique described and the effect of the Chinese health balls.

Our Nervous System

Man is an inquisitive creature. He is constantly looking for explanations for the phenomena he perceives. He wants to know everything about everything, and likes to fit what he knows into a system, so that it can be identified and placed in context.

Countless researchers have been concerned with understanding our nervous system, and the way in which external stimuli find their way inside and elicit a response. Thanks to, amongst others, the physicist Pavlov, who became famous for his research, we now have a very precise understanding of the laws governing the nervous system in the human body and its connecting, regulating function. Man is constantly exposed to external stimuli, and he is always – consciously or unconsciously – responding to these stimuli. The nervous system functions as the great connecting element in this, the link between the outer layer of the body and the organs, and between the organs themselves. In fact, the human body is a large cybernetic system, a network of automatically switching impulses and responses. Every organ affects every other organ, every organ reacts to every stimulus, every stimulus causes a bio-feedback of all the organs connected to the network.

The so-called 'holistic' healing method is based on this principle.

When an organ in our body becomes ill, a specific area of the skin, connected to that organ by nerves and delicate nerve endings, also reacts. The skin in that area becomes extra sensitive to pain. Conversely, it is possible to retrace the path to the affected organ from this skin reaction.

The man who discovered this, Head, described precisely which area

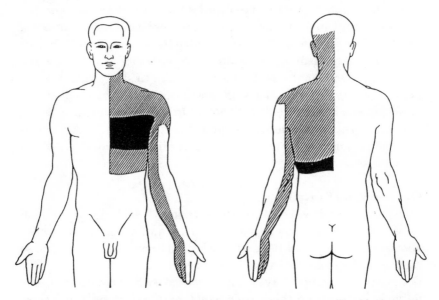

For heart conditions the areas of skin indicated here react. The black part is the actual area of pain, while the shaded parts indicate the area where there are vegetative and vaso-motoric reactions.

of skin corresponds with which organ. Therefore these areas are also known as Head zones, or the zones of Head. A more general name for these areas of reaction on the skin is: 'dermatoms'.

Thus, according to the results of Head's research, a disturbance in an internal organ causes an over-sensitive reaction in a dermatom connected with that organ. It is possible to influence the disturbed organ by means of special targeted stimulation of the same dermatom.

All these signals pass back and forth along the related part of the spinal cord. Along the entire spinal cord there are connections between the nerves, which run to the organs and the sensitive nerves with nerve endings on the surface of the skin. The spinal cord acts as a junction box between these two nerve circuits.

For example, we have known for a long time that a hot water bottle placed on a painful stomach often does not affect that organ with its heat directly. The sensitive nerves of the skin first pass on the heat stimulus to the spinal cord, from there the stimulus is passed onto the brain, and then it is passed back to the stomach via the spinal cord.

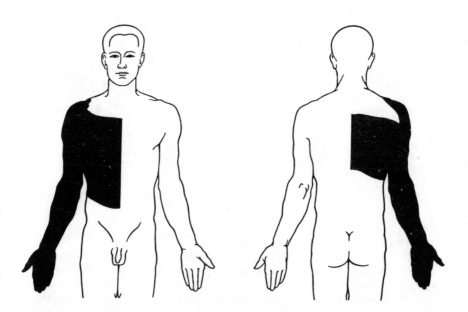

This shows the areas of the skin which become irritated when there is a disturbance in the lungs.

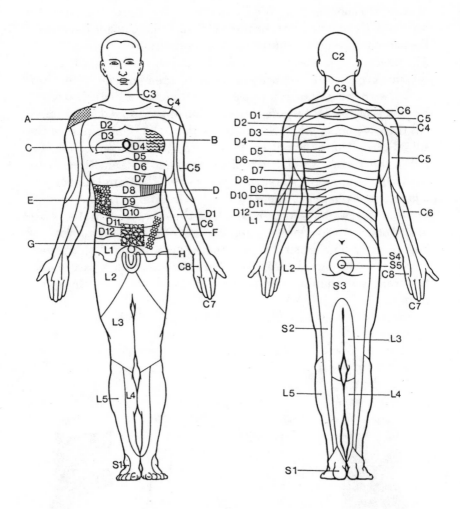

The Dermatoms According to Head

The skin is divided into a large number of strips, and each strip corresponds with an internal organ. The coding of the zones is linked to that of the spinal vertebrae. Each vertebra has a concentration of nerves which serves as a switch between the nerves of the dermatom and those of the organ. Here, the letter C indicates the cervical vertebrae, D the thoracic vertebrae, L the lumbar vertebrae, and S the caudal vertebrae, e.g., D4 = the first thoracic vertebra.

Organ Segments

Organ	Letter	Core area	Total zone
Diaphragm	A	C4	C4
Heart	B	D3,4	C3,4−D3-9
Stomach	C	D8	D7-9
Oesophagus	D	D4,5	D4-8
Liver, gall bladder	E	D8-11	C3-4,D7-11
Kidneys	F	D10-L1	D10-L2
Large intestine	G	D11-L1	D11-L1
Bladder	H	D11-L1	D11 L1

A number of therapies have been developed on the basis of Head's discoveries. For example, there are various methods of massage which are aimed at positively influencing the corresponding organs by treating the dermatoms. In so-called 'segment therapy', injections of procaine are given in a particular core area to influence disturbances in the related organ.

The natural medicine treatment method of giving injections in so-called 'pressure points' is also related to this. These pressure points were discovered by the doctor of natural medicine, Weihe, as areas, often no larger than a fingertip, which display a painful response in the case of complaints in the corresponding organs. Often the pain is only felt when pressure is put on these special points, but sometimes they can feel painful without being touched. Usually massaging the spot concerned, or simply pressing on it lightly, will remove the localized pain after a while, but it also has an effect on the corresponding organ.

'Locus-dolendi-acupuncture' is based on the same principle. The classical Chinese work on acupuncture, Huangdi Nei Ching, states: 'At the very place where the pain is felt, there is an acupuncture point.' Thus these points are often the core areas of the corresponding organs.

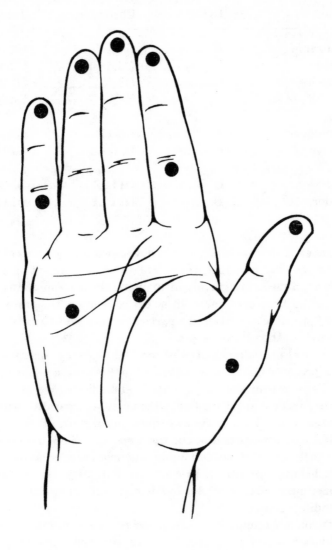

The most important acupuncture points on the inside of the hand are indicated above.

There are also dermatoms on the hands and feet, viz., the segments C6, C7 and C8, which means that the nerves in the hand have connections with the cervical vertebrae, which in turn connect with the aorta, the pituitary, the heart, the lungs and the bronchi. Therefore stimulating the inside of the hands should have an effect on these organs.

In Korea, a special type of acupuncture is practised which is based exclusively on the hands and reaches all the organs via a network of points.

Reflexology is a therapy which is well known in the West, and is based on the same principle of a reactive connection between the surface of the skin of the palms of the hands and the soles of the feet with all the organs in the body. By means of massage, or by using special foot rollers, the organs are affected through the skin, contributing in this way to an improvement in the condition of these organs, or even their recovery. Reflexology, which was developed by Carter, is often described as foot reflexology. This is because various organs are often 'affected' by means of a very thorough massage of the soles of the feet. But there are just as many areas on the hands, corresponding to most internal organs. A survey of these reflex zones on the hands is given on the next two pages.

Let us return to the health balls and the Chinese, who roll them around in the palms of their hands without apparently giving it any thought. The above description of dermatoms, pressure points and reflex zones shows that in fact the Chinese are certainly behaving in a meaningful way. By rotating the balls over the entire inside of their hands, they are massaging all the pressure points and zones, and thus, more or less, all their organs. This then, finally explains all those miraculous stories of positive results using the balls for such diverse complaints as problems with the spinal column, stomach ache, high blood pressure, heart disorders, intestinal complaints, nervousness etc. Suddenly these stories do not seem so strange any longer, for they are based on the same ancient tried and tested principles which underlie acupuncture and pressure point massage.

In addition, Chinese health balls have another positive side effect. As the balls are literally used with the hands, the muscles and the circulation of the hands, arms, neck and shoulders are stimulated. In this way the balls serve as a direct form of fitness training for this area.

Reflex Zones of the Hand

Left Hand

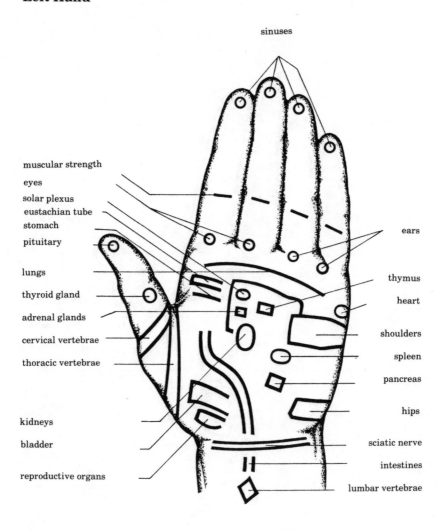

sinuses

muscular strength
eyes
solar plexus
eustachian tube
stomach
pituitary

ears

lungs

thymus

thyroid gland

heart

adrenal glands

cervical vertebrae

shoulders

thoracic vertebrae

spleen

pancreas

hips

kidneys

bladder

sciatic nerve

intestines

reproductive organs

lumbar vertebrae

Right hand

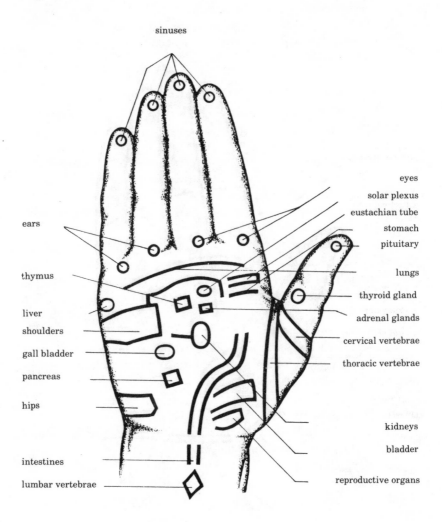

sinuses

eyes
solar plexus
eustachian tube
stomach
pituitary

ears

lungs

thymus

thyroid gland

liver

adrenal glands

shoulders

cervical vertebrae

gall bladder

thoracic vertebrae

pancreas

hips

kidneys

bladder

intestines

lumbar vertebrae

reproductive organs

All the areas and organs, the reflex zones of which are indicated on the preceding pages, are influenced by the use of Chinese health balls.

However, the ki meridians are also affected through the acupuncture points in the hand (e.g., the meridians of the heart, lung, circulation of the blood, and the large and small intestine). It is this effect that has given the balls another name, for they are sometimes known as 'meridian balls'.

Summary

If we list the most important facts mentioned up to this point, we arrive at the following summary:

1. The life force, known as 'ki' runs through the body via the ki meridians. There are a number of centres along these meridians which are sometimes called 'acupuncture points'.
2. Disruptions of the internal organs cause reactions on the surface of the body.
3. Every organ has its own corresponding zone, which is sometimes far removed from the related organ.
4. It is possible to influence the corresponding organ by treating these so-called reflex zones.
5. The reflex zones for a large number of organs can be found on the feet, as well as the hands.
6. Chinese health balls work on all the reflex zones and acupuncture points on the insides of the hands, and therefore on all the meridians and organs related to these.

Kirlian Photography

The effect of the balls can be measured by different methods. Changes in the energy level can be shown by means of electro- acupuncture or Kirlian photography. The changes in the heat that is radiated can be measured by thermography, EC, EEG, and by measuring the blood pressure. An increase in the heat that is radiated indicates an improvement in the circulation.

On the next page, Kirlian photography is used to show the results on the left hand before and after thirty minutes with Chinese health balls.

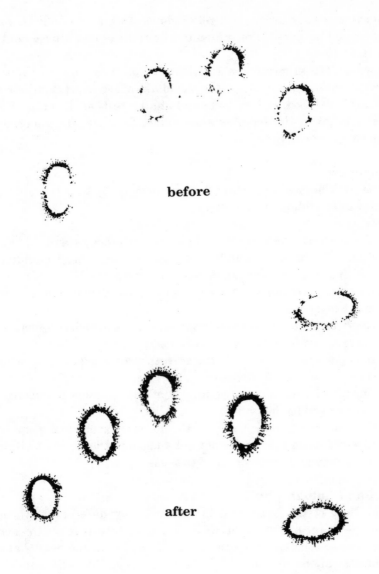

before

after

The five fingertips of the left hand are shown above, before and after thirty minutes of exercising with meridian balls. Clearly the energy radiation is stronger below. The energy level of the body has obviously improved.

Muscles and Blood Circulation
In order to roll the balls around the palm of the hand, it is necessary to stretch out the hand and bend the arm slightly. This movement means that the bending muscles are constantly engaged. The hand and fingers move incessantly as the balls roll round, so that the muscles of the hand and the wrist joint are trained.

In the hand there is a finely branched network of capillaries and nerves. The stimulation of this network by the balls rolling around is transferred to the larger blood vessels and nerves of the hand, and in turn, to those of the arm. The lymphatic vessels are activated, and the tendons and joints become suppler.

The metabolic process in the tissue of the hand is stimulated to greater activity, resulting in a faster removal of metabolic waste products.

The constant movement of the fingers is converted into muscular movements of the lower and upper arm. It is well known that exercising the muscles promotes the circulation of the blood, on the one hand, because the movement of the muscles massages the blood vessels, and on the other hand, because more fuel (i.e., oxygen) is required, and the blood flows more quickly to supply sufficient oxygen. As a result, it is not only in the arm that is used that the circulation is stronger, but the circulation improves throughout the body because of the stronger pumping action and the faster supply and removal of blood via the heart.

The constant movement of the muscles, which is transferred through the lower and upper arm up to the shoulder girdle, also affects the muscles in the neck. You can discover this for yourself: place the fingers of your right hand in the curve on the left side of your neck on the cervical muscle, and then clench your left fist – you will feel the cervical muscle constricting.

The balls come in three sizes. (We will come back to discuss in detail the various sorts and sizes in a later chapter.) The smallest size of ball weighs approximately 330 grammes per pair, the average size 460 grammes and the largest size, approximately 580 grammes. Because of their weight, they have the same effect on the muscles of the arm, shoulder and chest as small dumbbells. When you are exercising with the balls, this is a light form of weight training: the above-mentioned muscles gradually become noticeably stronger as a result of the double effect of weight plus movement.

All the muscles of the body form an enclosed system. Certain schools of natural medicine, and other therapies which are aimed at dealing with muscular problems and correcting the motor system, do not treat only the problem area, but often start making corrections in a completely different place. For example, for a disturbance in the area of the cervical vertebrae, treatment often begins with the muscles in the foot, and then slowly moves up through the muscles in the leg. There is the well-known example of support soles to relieve headaches: collapsed muscles in the feet influence the whole muscular structure, and therefore the position of the spinal column, which in turn affects the circulation of the blood and the unrestricted functioning of the nervous system.

The subtle effect of Chinese health balls on the muscular system and the circulation of the blood can in the long term achieve results varying from a relief of neck complaints to an improvement of a dull feeling in the legs. It is particularly the very light stimulation produced by the balls that encourages the body to become active itself. In the end, it is always the body itself, stimulated, helped and activated by whatever therapy, that heals itself.

The use of Chinese health balls can certainly be called a therapy, although it is not a therapy from which one can expect rapid results. If you wish to achieve results with the balls, you must have patience above all − long-term patience, because it is a long time before there are any really noticeable results, and short-term patience, because you must set aside time every day for some quiet exercise with the balls. The word 'manipulation', which is sometimes used for a method which is used to help restore us to health, is based on the Latin word 'manus' or hand; the hand, the part of the body involved in touch, contact, warmth. When you are using Chinese health balls, you are manipulating in the true sense of the word: you are making contact with yourself, and taking the time to become aware of your own body and the reactions of your body. Working with the balls is like a meditation exercise: you are very quietly concentrating on one thing, in complete peace. When you have sat for a while rolling the balls, you will notice that all thoughts slowly ebb away, and you start to feel an inner tranquillity. This in itself is a positive result of exercizing with the balls. It relaxes and calms not only the vegetative nervous system, but also the mind.

Thus, the balls work into two ways. On the one hand, they activate and stimulate a large number of body functions (which means that they are very suitable, for example, for older people to remain fit in a way which does not require too much effort); on the other hand, they have a calming and relaxing effect, so that they have been able to achieve good results when used by restless, nervous people. Children with concentration problems can sometimes benefit from exercising with the balls. Often they like to 'play' with the chiming balls, while this 'play' has a regulating effect on their powers of co-ordination and concentration. Good results have been achieved in this way in China, where the balls originate.

Brainhemispheres

The so-called P.E.T. scanner is used to measure the activity of the brain. Tests with this scanner have shown that when the right hand is active, the activity in the left half of the brain increases, and vice versa: when the left hand is active, there is an increase in activity in the right half of the brain. This brings us to another interesting possibility of Chinese health balls: the specific training of the two halves of the brain. By now, it is well known that the western educational and learning system mainly trains the half of the brain which deals with analytical and rational functions. For most people, this is the left half of the brain. The other half of the brain governs the intuitive functions, and operates in relationships instead of in separate units. It is often assumed that, in general, Asians operate more on the basis of this second half of the brain (i.e., usually the right half).

However this may be, when the emphasis in development is only on one half of the brain, the development can never be truly harmonious and balanced.

Various different methods and exercises have been developed to train the so-called 'non-dominant' half of the brain. Chinese health balls are certainly another good method. Kinesiological muscle tests can be used to determine which half of the brain is dominant in a person. The hand which corresponds with this half of the brain is on the other side of the body. Therefore by training the other hand intensively with the balls, the other half of the brain is also stimulated to become more active.

Sound

The metal balls are hollow inside. A second smaller ball rolls round inside it, constantly striking against a small metal flap which starts to vibrate, and therefore produces a sound. In a pair of balls which go together, one ball produces a yin tone, the other a yang tone. It is a scientifically known fact that the ear is connected to all the nerves in the body, and communicates with all the parts of the body and all the organs via these nerves. Sound has a great effect on people: just think of the reaction to chalk scratching on a blackboard, or the use of 'musak' in shopping centres to encourage people to buy, marching music which inspires soldiers to fight. These are negative examples of the influence which sounds have on the human organism. Fortunately there are also sounds which have a positive effect. The sounds which are produced by Chinese health balls belong to the latter category.

The importance of the ear and the impulses which it transmits to the whole human organism is clear from the fact that by the middle of pregnancy the embryo's inner ear and organ of balance are completely developed, and all the nerve connections with these organs have been formed. From this time the embryo can receive sounds from outside, while still in the womb. These impulses from the outside world have a stimulating effect on the development of the embryo's brain and whole body.

The organ of balance not only regulates the body's orientation in space and the co-ordination of movement in space, but also influences a number of vegetative functions.

The cochlea in the inner ear is responsible for our sense of hearing. The organ of balance and the cochlea are interconnected by the liquid in the inner ear. Fine hair cells register impulses of both sound and movement, transmitting both to the cerebral cortex and to the various parts of the body and organs in the form of electro-chemical impulses.

Thus, the effect of the yin and yang sounds of Chinese health balls reaches every part of the body through the ear. It is not only the pleasant sound which has a harmonizing and relaxing effect, it is the frequency of the sound itself which softly vibrates in all the organs and parts of the body along the nerve channels via the organs of hearing and balance.

A Summary of Effects

At the end of this chapter on the effects of Chinese health balls, we would like to list all the factors which play a part. These factors are:

1. **Vibration**
   The soft vibration acts as a relaxing stimulus which has a deep effect on the tissues. The circulation of the blood and the lymph are stimulated and the nerve fibres are calmed.

2. **Pressure**
   The pressure exerted by the balls acts as a massage, making the tissue more supple, and activating the whole circulation by means of its pumping action.

3. **Heat**
   The activity of the muscles produces heat, not only in localized areas, but throughout the body, by means of a kinetic effect. This heat activates the internal organs, and at the same time expands the blood vessels so that circulation is improved.
   Heat also has a calming effect on the nerves.

4. **Sound**
   Sound simultaneously has a calming and invigorating, relaxing and stimulating effect.

5. **Isometric effect**
   The weight of the balls strengthens the muscles of the hand and arm.

All in all, the Chinese health balls are tangible proof of the fact that an apparently simple phenomenon can have many different explanations.

Part 3

Varieties

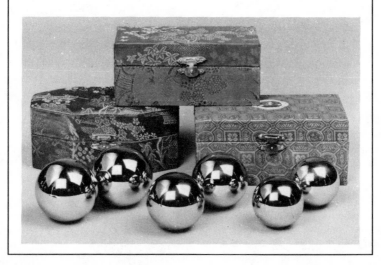

The Range

When you go to a shop to buy a set of Chinese health balls, you will often be confronted with a variety of different sorts. Each to his own, you might think, but the question is: what exactly do you want? And which are the best to buy?
To help you answer this question, the following chapter gives a survey of the range of balls, most of which are available in the United States.

This chapter contains a number of starting points which are important for making the right choice.

Whatever material they are made of, the balls mostly come in one of these sizes: small, medium or large. The normal metal balls come in two additional smaller sizes.

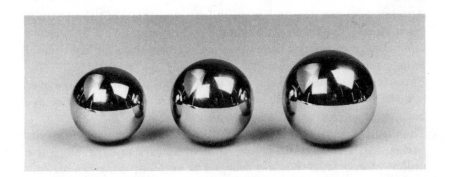

A Survey

In the United States, various different sorts of balls are available in shops which also sell other Asian (art) products. We begin our survey with the most common types, which are illustrated on the next page. This is followed by a number of other types, which may not be available or may be very rare, and which we have therefore not illustrated, but which we have included in the survey for the sake of completeness.

Illustrated Types

1. *The normal metal balls*

These balls are available in five sizes. The smallest size has a diameter of 3.5 cm. and weighs ± 165 grammes per pair. They are suitable for children who like to have a try. Next size is 4 cm. in diameter, and weighs ± 222 grammes per pair. These balls fit into the hands of older children and small adults. Balls with a diameter of 4.5 cm. and a weight of 330 grammes per pair are also suitable for people with small hands as well as for beginners of all sizes. People with some experience can move on to a bigger size: 5 cm. in diameter with a weight of ± 460 grammes per pair.

Finally, there is the largest size, 5.5 cm. in diameter, with a weight of approximately 580 grammes per pair. These balls are suitable for people who have learnt to use the other balls without any difficulty, and who are now interested in a more intensive effect – and for people with large hands !

2. *Marble, stone and jade balls*

These balls are solid and do not produce any sound. Thus they are a solution for people who do not like the clinking sound of the metal balls.

Another advantage for some users is that because of the nature of the material, the surface is slightly rougher, and the balls therefore offer a better grip. In addition, they feel warmer than the 'cold' metal balls, particularly at first.

These balls – especially the jade variety, but also the marble ones available in various different shades – are a delight to the eye because of their attractive appearance.

The disadvantage of this type of ball is that after lengthy use, the surface can become rougher as a result of friction, and therefore also duller. Moreover, if they are dropped by accident, they can break.

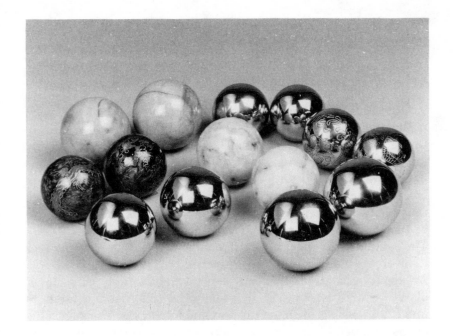

jade   smooth metal (small)

cloisonné   marble   engraved metal

smooth metal (medium)   smooth metal (large)

The most common size for these balls is the medium size, although they are also available in the large and small sizes. Their weight, depending on the type of stone, is approximately the same or slightly less than that of a standard metal ball of the same diameter.

3. Engraved metal balls

A phoenix is depicted on the yin ball, a dragon on the yang ball. In China, the phoenix is the symbol of resurrection, renewal and immortality; the dragon is the symbol of matter, the spirit and the male principle. It is traditional to give gifts depicting these two symbols to a couple who are getting married, as an expression of the wish that the two partners will henceforth form one harmonious entity, be successful and enjoy eternal happiness.

The same wish is engraved on the balls: may the person who uses them create a unity from the contrasts which he experiences.

An apparent contradiction can turn out to be a unity on a higher plane. Anyone who learns to understand this, has mastered an important basic principle of success and happiness. The engraving on the balls gives an opportunity of reflecting on this thought, and in this way reminds the user that the balls are not only a physical training method, but can also be an effective factor in training consciousness.

However, the engraved lines also have a physical effect. The slight unevenness of the design on the smooth surface of the ball produces extra friction with the skin, and therefore a more intensive effect on the skin's reflex zones.

4. Cloisonné balls

Because of their beautiful appearance, cloisonné balls could be called the thoroughbreds of Chinese health balls. However, like thoroughbreds, they are almost too delicate for everyday use. They have the disadvantage which stone balls also have: they are easily damaged. On the other hand, they also have a number of advantages in common with stone balls: because they have a slightly rougher surface, they lie more securely in the hand and they feel 'warmer' than the ordinary smooth metal balls. The rough surface has the advantage of the engraved balls: a more intensive effect on the reflex zones of the skin.

Cloisonné balls are always hollow, but do not always contain an element of sound.

These brilliantly coloured balls are an example of the influence of Emperor Kwan Long of the Ching Dynasty, who elevated the balls to the level of objets d'art. They are decorated in a variety of ways; in some cases the motif of the dragon and the phoenix is used. The balls with a sound element can be used like ordinary Chinese health balls, but it is advisable to use them very carefully. The completely hollow balls which do not produce a sound are really used only as objets d'art.

Types of Balls Which Are Not Illustrated
5. Balls for children
These are normal Chinese health balls, but in a very small size, specially adapted for children's hands, with a diameter of 4 cm. and a weight of approximately 250 grammes per pair.

6. Musical balls
In fact, these balls cannot really be considered to be Chinese health balls, because their effect is based exclusively on sound. They are small balls with a diameter of between 19 and 35 mm. They are not used in pairs, but individually, and are made of gold or silver. They are rolled in the palm of the hand, or worn on a chain around the neck.

The special characteristic of these balls is that when they are moved, they produce a chord composed of 28 notes. This mantra sound has a harmonious effect on the body and the soul. The so-called 'yin-yang ball', which is made of black brass engraved with the yin-yang symbol, which produces an equally beautiful sound, is related to these balls.

As noted above, the therapeutic value of these balls lies only in the sound they produce. The weight is too negligible to have any effect. In between these balls and ordinary Chinese health balls, there is another type of ball which is fairly small in size, and is used in the same way as ordinary Chinese health balls, but is distinct from them because of the special sound, which is reminiscent of true musical balls.

7. Balls with a special appearance
Apart from stone balls, engraved balls and cloisonné balls, there are three other types which are distinguished by an exceptionally beautiful appearance.

The first type which deserves a mention in this category is the gold coloured ball. This is no different from the ordinary Chinese health ball, except that it is a gold rather than a silver colour. Gold is associated with yin; silver with yang. Gold coloured balls are usually medium-sized.

The second sort in this category is the black ball. This ball has a warm, velvety surface with a brilliant, matt anthracite colour.

The last type to be mentioned is the lacquered ball. First, the surface is painted with a design, and then a protective layer of lacquer is applied over it.

8. Magnetic balls
Small magnets are placed in the surface of these balls, which have the same magnetizing effect as, for example, magnetic bracelets.

Variations on a Theme
To conclude this list of different balls, we will mention a few variations which have only recently been developed, and which look like
Chinese health balls, although in two of the three cases, they have
little in common with the true balls.

9. Bubble balls
These balls are made of an elastic, synthetic material and are 7 cm.
in diameter. One ball is used at a time. As its name suggests, the surface of this ball is covered with conical protrutions. You try to
squeeze and knead the ball in the palm of the hand to work on the
reflex zones. There are even larger sizes which are specially made for
exercises with the feet.

10. Twin balls
In this variation, two Chinese health balls are joined together with
a bar, to make a sort of dumbbell. In fact, they are used as dumbbells
by groups practising Tai Chi or QiGong in gymnastic exercises,
dance exercises and exercises for the wrist. Often they are used by
groups. The effect of the combination of sounds that is produced
gives a very special dimension to the exercises.

11. The lemniscate
A track wide enough for the ball to roll along is made on an oblong
board in the shape of a figure of eight. You hold the board sideways
on in front of you, letting the ball roll round and round the figure of
eight (lemniscate), following it with your eyes. This is a way of training your powers of concentration, the co-ordination of the eyes, and
the two halves of the brain, and it relaxes the cervical muscles as the
head moves to and fro. Anyone who is good with their hands can
make the board themselves. The width should be such that when the
figure of eight shape has been made, the board is comfortable to hold,
with the hands stretched out and elbows bent. The figure of eight can
be carved or chiselled, and sanded, or it can be made by gluing cur-
ved strips of wood, synthetic material, or (corrugated) cardboard
onto the board.

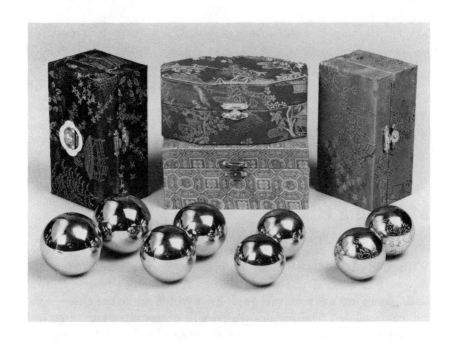

When you choose a set of balls for your own personal use, your choice should not only be based on what is most useful, but you should let your personal preference play a role as well.

Making a Choice

With such a large variety available, it may seem difficult to make a choice. However, if you would like to start using Chinese health balls, there are a few simple guidelines which make the choice considerably easier. The factors which will determine your selection can actually be divided into two categories: the size and the way in which the balls are made.

Size
It is obvious to imagine that you should choose the size of the balls corresponding to the size of the hand which will use them. This is certainly one way of choosing, but there is one objection. When you first start to exercise with Chinese health balls, you notice that using them is by no means always easy. Practice always makes perfect, but you surely will have to practise a little before you even acquire some basic dexterity. You will find that with the hand you use least (i.e., the left hand for right-handed people, and the right hand for left-handed people), it will take quite a while before you can roll the balls around without any problems.

Thus, if you start straightaway with quite large-sized balls, it will be even more difficult. In other words, the smaller the balls, the easier it is to learn to use them.

For this reason, beginners are always advised to start with the smallest sized balls. The shape of your hand does not really play a part in this. Whether you have a small or a large hand, it is a matter of first acquiring some dexterity. It is even conceivable that a small, supple and/or muscular hand will learn to master the balls more quickly than a large, coarse hand which has had little training, even though the larger palm of the hand provides more support for the balls so that they do not slip out of the hand so easily.

Therefore, start with small balls and do not give up when you cannot seem to get the hang of it at first. Persevere patiently, practise a little everyday, and you'll find that eventually it will become quite automatic.

Once you have achieved this, and the balls roll around automatically so that you have no difficulty with any of the exercises with the balls, the time is ripe to change to a larger size. The difference in size and weight of these larger balls forms a new challenge in itself, and also makes for a more intense effect. Because of its weight, the larger ball has a deeper effect on the reflex zones, the pressure points and the muscles of the hand. The muscles themselves have to work harder; in addition, the sound of the larger balls is also heavier and has a different effect on the body and the mind.

Therefore, to summarize with regard to size, we would advise you to start with balls which are as small as possible; once you have acquired a certain degree of dexterity, use the largest possible balls for the best possible results.

Obviously this does not mean that you will have to buy larger balls immediately when you've had the smaller ones for a while, or that you have to throw away the smaller ones once you have actually made the decision to buy larger balls.

You can also work very well with the smaller balls in the long term − by devoting more time to the exercises and by doing a greater variety of exercises, you will still achieve good results.

If you buy larger balls after using smaller ones, you also acquire the possibility to exercise with four or even more balls at the same time: with three, four or five balls in one hand or with both hands simultaneously, and a number of balls in each hand.

This last exercise is an exceptionally good exercise for your powers of concentration and co-ordination. It is easiest to use balls of the same size; if you have balls of different sizes, you can either divide the sizes equally between both hands, or use the heaviest balls with the hand that has the most dexterity.

Variety

Chinese health balls of different makes are imported to our country from China. Like any product in the world, there are small differences between them.

In the case of the smooth metal balls, these are differences in the material and the sound. This does not mean that some balls are not as good as others. It merely means that there may be a distinction, so that what is considered pleasant by one person may be slightly less agreeable to another. Therefore it is important to let yourself be guided by your own feelings and to choose the balls which feel right in your own hands, have a nice tocuh and a pleasant sound.

With regard to marble, jade and stone balls, the choice is even more personal.

We have remarked before, that some people do not like the tinkling sound of the metal balls; for them balls made of a variety of stone are therefore a good choice. These balls also feel different from metal balls; the choice between the two materials is a matter of pure personal preference. Some people choose stone balls just for their appearance: they find them more attractive than the shiny, mirror-like, metal balls and choose a particular colour which satisfies their own sense of beauty.

Engraved balls and cloisonné balls are often chosen for purely aesthetic reasons. If you actually want to use them as well for the exercises, it is a good idea, when you are in the shop, to roll them in the palm of your hand for a while with your eyes shut. What does that feel like ? Are you sure the irregularities in the surface are not irritating ? If this is the case, do not buy the balls to work with them. Buy them as decorative objects, place them in a good spot so you can enjoy looking at them everyday and buy smooth balls to work with.

All balls, of every variety, are supplied in a little box lined with embroidered silk (on the outside) and velvet (on the inside) with special recesses in the bottom into which the balls fit exactly, depending on their size. This box is also the best place to keep them.

Maintenance

The balls are stored like treasure in the little box in which they are sold. If you want to enjoy your balls for a long time, then you should handle them carefully, as though they were real treasures.

At first it's a good idea to rub them with a soft cloth whenever you've used them, and then to replace them in their box. Don't simply leave them lying around; before you know where you are, they'll roll around and fall, and this can cause all sorts of problems.

When you exercise with the balls, make sure that they don't bump into each other, but remain in constant flowing contact with each other as they roll around. This prevents them from being scratched and dented.

The balls will benefit if you occasionally polish them with some good quality oil, such as sewing machine oil or linseed oil, or with a little bit of vaseline. Make sure that you rub them thoroughly afterwards so that no oil remains.

Because of the constant contact with the skin of the palms of your hand, the balls are gradually covered with a layer of grease from your skin mixed with crystals of perspiration. This layer, which cannot be removed by polishing the balls with oil, has a chemical composition which eventually affects the surface of the balls. To prevent this, you can occasionally wash the balls with a mild washing-up liquid. Afterwards, they should be thoroughly rinsed under running water so that there are no remnants of the detergent, and then they should be carefully rubbed dry. Then treat them as above, with oil or vaseline. You will particularly have to clean them in this way if you have sweaty palms.

If you lend the balls to anyone else, rinse and polish them as well, to remove both the layer that may have formed, and the remnants of the other user's energy.

It won't hurt the balls to come into contact with water but it's certainly not a good idea to leave them lying in it ! In addition, avoid contact with other substances and liquids such as perfumes, acids, mineral salts, etc.

Part 4

Exercises

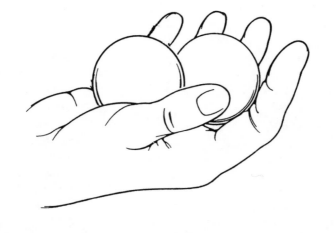

General Practice

Now that the effect has been explained, and you have made a choice from the range of balls available, it's time to actually start using them. There are a large number of exercises in the next section of the book, and these will help you to explore the various possibilities of the balls for yourself. Think of the exercises as a source of encouragement and inspiration. They give an impression of the various possibilities, but they certainly should not be considered as rigid rules which must be carried out in exactly the way described and in the order in which they appear.

Therefore, start by reading through the exercises at your leisure, choose the ones which appeal to you, and above all, use them as a basis for exploring, feeling, experimenting, playing. The more serious and patient you are when you practice, the better your chance of good results — but this seriousness only applies to the extent to which you are prepared to persevere. It is certainly not the intention that you enter into an obsessive battle for results in which the balls become your opponents. Enjoy, play and feel — that's the best way of persevering for a long time and therefore the best way for successful results!

Once Again, Yin and Yang

In a set of balls, one always represents yin, the other yang; therefore one ball produces a yin sound, the other a yang sound. The only way of being sure which ball produces which sound is to look at balls with pictures of a dragon and a phoenix: the dragon is the yang ball, the phoenix is the yin.

Yin and yang together produce a perfect equilibrium: therefore, when you work with both balls at the same time, you can never give yourself more yin or more yang.

Or at least that's what you might think. But because one person has a stronger yin and needs yang, while the opposite might apply to someone else, techniques have been developed which enable us to generate more yin or yang as we choose, so that we can in this way achieve an equilibrium in our own yinyang balance. To start with, it is necessary to know whether your constitution is more yin or more yang. In order to establish this, there are a number of identification points which we will describe here.

The yin constitution
The yin type is to a greater or lesser extent predominantly introverted, calm, sensitive, passive, silent with an artistic temperament. Physically this type has a soft, round shape sometimes tending to weakness. The upper eyelid covers the top half of the pupil. This type often feels cold and has a great need for warmth. Therefore, the favourite food is usually cooked food and it certainly has to be hot.

The yang constitution
The yang type is more or less extrovert, active, rational with a practical inclination, physical and analytical. Physically this person is often powerful, sturdy and sometimes sinewy. The upper part of the pupil is visible while the lower half is often partially covered by the lower eyelid. This type has a great deal of inner warmth. Raw food is often the favourite and is certainly very suitable because it neutralizes the excessive heat.

On the basis of these short and therefore rather simple guidelines, it is still possible to establish what sort of person you are. In many cases, the emphasis is not clearly on one side or the other, because every person is a combination of types. However, sometimes it is clear that the balance is weighted on one side and in this case, corrective exercises are particularly appropriate.

In fact, the exercises are not so much specifically aimed at restoring the balance − it's rather the way in which the exercise is carried out which determines whether it has a yin or a yang influence. Therefore, all the exercises, especially the simpler ones, can be performed as yin or yang exercises. The distinction is made by differences in speed, direction and the length of time the balls are rotated.

Exercises for strengthening the yin force
1. Speed: allow the balls to rotate slowly; the more slowly, the better. Make sure that the rotating movement is always a flowing movement.
2. Direction: rotate the balls to the right, i.e., in a clockwise direction. This movement is considered as a yin movement, whether it is drawn with the arms through the air, walked, danced or carried out in any other way.
3. Length of time: rotating balls for a short time strengthens the yin force. The balls are cold when you start and that is yin. The cold balls attract heat, which is yang, from the body. To make sure that the effect strengthens the yin force, you should stop before the balls are heated up and put them away until they are cold again.

Exercises for strengthening the yang force
1. Speed: the faster the balls are rotated the more yang is generated. Again it is important that the rotating movement is a flowing movement and that the balls do not start flying around and colliding with each other.
2. Direction: to the left, an anti-clockwise movement is a yang movement.
3. Length of time: If the balls are left in the hand for a long time and are rotated they become warmer. The heat which is stored in the ball in this way is returned to the body and adds yang force. The combination of rotating the balls quickly and for a long time generates a considerable amount of heat, i.e., yang force.

To summarize, it could be said that working slowly and for a short time is yin, while working quickly for a long time is yang. Using this simple technique, you can do more than merely affect your physical balance. Regardless of your own basic constitution, if you feel the need at any particular time for introspection and contemplation, you can achieve this by slowly rotating the balls to the right with interruptions. If you need a surge of energy or want to stimulate your activity, rotate the balls quickly to the left until you can clearly feel the heat flowing through your body. Therefore it may be advisable too to do a yang exercise in the morning to become active and a yin exercise in the evening to relax.

The Basic Exercise

In this book we have mentioned several times that the balls are rotated in the palm of the hand. This movement is the basis for all the other exercises; if you want to start working with the balls, you have to start by mastering this movement.

As we advised before, you should start with small balls. In most cases you will find it difficult enough to keep the balls in the palm of your hand, even if they aren't very large.

Because of this sort of problem which a beginner may have, it is a good idea to make sure that you start exercising over a soft surface. Sit down somewhere where there is a soft carpet on the floor or put some cushions or a blanket around you. You can also practise over a table covered with a soft cloth or blanket. At first, the balls are almost bound to fall a few times. Metal balls may be dented and stone balls can crack. If you continue to use stone balls when they have been damaged, this can also lead to scratches or dents on the other ball, even if it is not damaged itself.

However, even if you drop the balls at first, and even if you can hardly get any movement with balls in the beginning, let alone a 'flowing rotating movement' – do not despair. Starting is always difficult, your fingers have not yet become adept. Try it for a little while every day and you'll notice that you soon start to improve.

In many people the co-ordination between the muscles in the hand and those of the arms and corresponding parts of the brain is by no means as good as it might be. At first, you may have to think very deeply about every movement of the fingers before you can make the balls roll about at all. But gradually it will become easier until you can manage to rotate the balls automatically, without thinking about it. When you've arrived at this stage, remember how much you have already achieved and to what extent the delicate motor co-ordination of your hands, as well as the above mentioned brain-muscle co-ordination, has progressed ! Once you've got this far, you'll notice that you'll not only be able to work the balls with your hands held out, but that you can rotate them with your hands in any position. Playing with the balls in this way, you'll discover more and more possibilities and variations for yourself.

The Basic Exercise - Step by Step

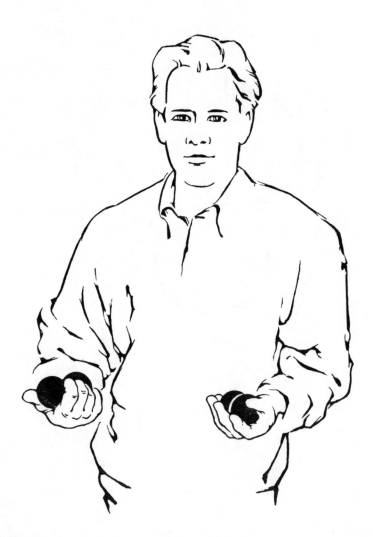

First step

You can stand up, or sit down. Make sure that your arms and particularly your elbows and lower arms are quite free. Start by holding the balls in your most dexterous hand. Later on you can also practice with the other hand or with both hands at once.

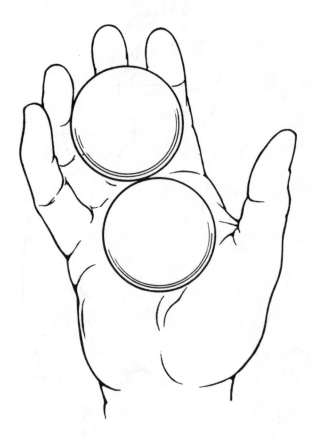

Second step

In the starting position, one of the balls lies in the middle of the palm of the hand, while the other ball is above this, resting on the middle finger and the ring finger. All the fingers are slightly bent, and the thumb, little finger and index finger are held a bit higher so that the balls remain in place.

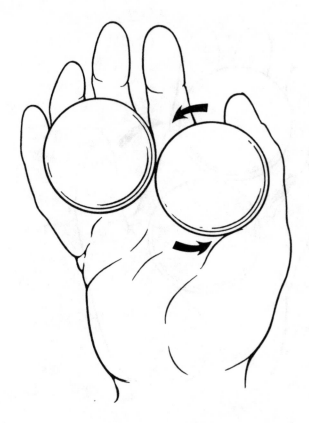

Third step
Lower the little finger slightly and at the same time raise the index finger, middle finger and ring finger. This will make the upper ball move towards the little finger and down, pushing the ball which was in the palm of the hand towards the thumb.

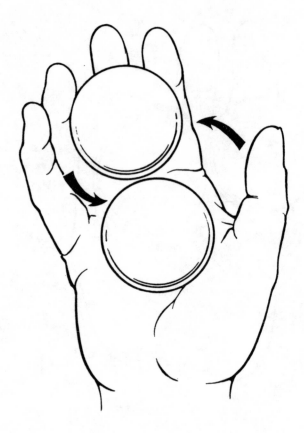

Fourth step

Press one ball down with the little finger at the same time as pressing the other ball sideways and up with the thumb. The two balls have now changed places, or in other words, you have carried out half of the rotation movement.

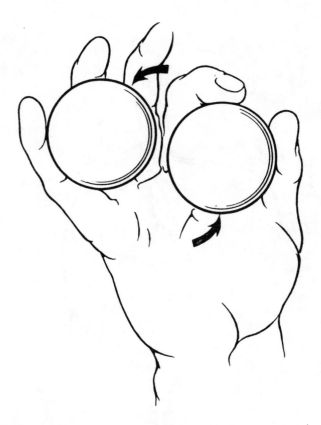

Fifth step

Hold the index finger, middle finger and ring finger at right angles to the palm of the hand as far as possible. As a result, the balls keep rolling along these three fingers from the thumb to the little finger, and the thumb gives them a little push upwards, while the little finger pushes them back down and back to the thumb. The faster this movement is made, the better the rotation of the balls keeps going. After some practice, the hand also starts to move in a single flowing movement, so that the heel of the thumb, with the thumb on one side and the little finger on the other, keeps the movement going and defines it.

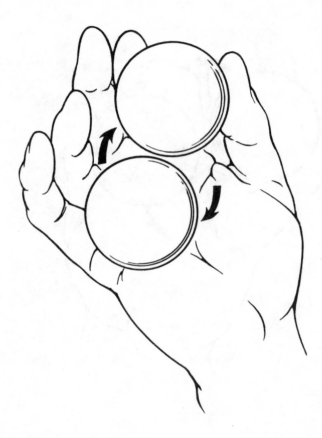

Sixth step

Once you've mastered this rotation in an anti-clockwise direction, it is time to try it in a clockwise direction. This time you lower the index finger and the ring finger slightly from their starting position (second step), and then raise the little finger and the heel of the thumb slightly, so that the upper ball rolls down to the thumb and the lower one to the little finger. By slightly bending first the index finger, and then the thumb, you consecutively give the balls a little push in that direction, and the rotating movement really gets going.

For most people it's easiest to rotate the balls in an anticlockwise direction with the left hand, and in a clockwise direction with the right hand. This is because of the shape of the hand; the balls simply roll more easily via the thumb and the heel of the thumb to the wrist than to the fingers. This means that the circle they describe is larger, so that the balls move more quickly and the rotating movement is continued automatically. Therefore, start by practising the movement which you find easiest, and then try the other movement until you've mastered this as well.

At first, the balls will collide with each other quite a bit and move through your hands in a rather awkward way. However, gradually you'll notice the movement becomes more even. Your fingers become more supple and you acquire greater dexterity, so finally, the balls roll around in an elegant, flowing movement through your hands, constantly in contact with each other. It's good to remember that the exercises and the description of the movements given here are meant only to help you. You'll soon notice for yourself how you can move the balls best, and develop your own method. With normal practice it's advisable to continue until the balls have been thoroughly warmed up and your fingers have lost any stiffness they may have had in the beginning. The longer and the more often you work with the balls, the sooner you'll become aware of good results. This is easier to achieve than it seems: you don't have to set any time aside to use the balls. I practise for an hour or two almost every day and use the time when my hands have nothing else to do anyway: when I'm thinking about a problem, when I'm watching television, or even when I'm taking a walk. (N.B. You can only do this when you've really mastered the technique. If you're not quite sure, it's best to continue practising at home on the carpet, because if you drop them there they won't become damaged. Out on the street, they'll certainly break if you drop them by accident.) When I feel restless before going to sleep, I rotate the balls for a while to relax. I can recommend it as a perfect remedy for sleeping!

Not everyone will want to work with Chinese health balls regularly for a long time. Some people might only wish to use them occasionally as a way of calming down, to play with, or to spend a few idle minutes in an agreeable way.

However, if you wish to use them to improve your general health, you will certainly have to spend ten minutes practising every day.

This is the only way in which you'll really benefit from the various ways in which the balls work.

Once you've completely mastered the basic exercise, you can start to do other exercises instead, or as well. You can invent these exercises yourself or pursue the different possibilities which are mentioned later in this book. For example, one very simple exercise is to do the ordinary basic movements in both directions and with both hands, at the same time or one after the other – but with your hands behind your back ! You'll need more dexterity and concentration to do this, and the greater demands you put on your powers of concentration and co-ordination, the more you'll stimulate the central nervous system. Before we describe a whole range of possible exercises, we'll give a few general hints to help the exercises to be as beneficial and effective as possible.

First of all, try to relax and breathe deeply. This is not so much a matter of monitoring your breathing, but more of being aware of the fact that you're breathing in a relaxed manner. In this way, your breathing is automatically regulated in a deep and calm tempo.

Secondly, when you notice that the muscles of your hand and/or arm become tired, stop using that hand. You could work with the other hand for a while, but rest the tired muscles until they've recovered. Don't force them in any way and trust in your body's reactions.

Thirdly, when you notice that your muscles become tired for longer, or even that you're in pain, stop using the balls for a few days. In general, using the balls cannot adversely affect health. However, if you notice that a complaint for which you want to use the balls is getting worse, wait a while and consult your doctor, a physiotherapist or a reliable alternative healer, preferably with experience of working with ki, if you don't recover your normal health soon.

Exercises

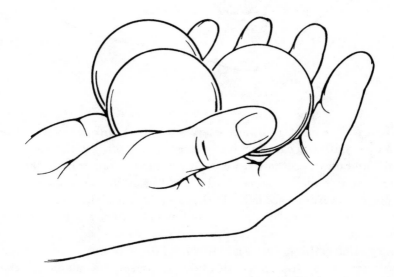

With Three Balls

This exercise is carried out with three balls, starting by using the smallest size. Take them in the palm of your hand and work with them in the same way as you would with two balls. The important difference is that the hand and the fingers must be spread further apart and held flatter, so that there's room for the three balls. The thumb pushes one of the balls around, while the little finger ensures that the two other balls move along with it.

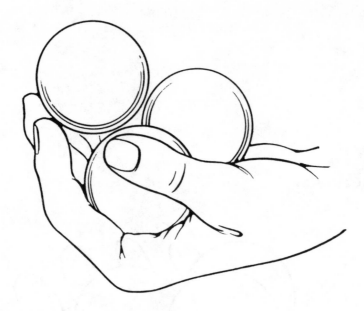

When you've mastered these exercises in both directions with the smallest ball, you can start using larger balls. Start with two small balls and one medium-sized ball. If you have large hands, you can then use two medium-sized balls, and finally you can progress to using all medium-sized balls. In this exercise the same applies as for any other exercise: the greater the level of difficulty, the stronger the effect.

A variation of this exercise is to lift one of the balls over the other two each time. To do this, alternately take the ball on the outside and the one on the inside (see illustration).

With Four Balls

This exercise is best carried out with the smallest sized balls. If you have very large hands, you could eventually replace one of the balls by a medium-sized ball; the largest size is certainly not suitable for this exercise.

Again, start by placing the balls in the palm of your hand. Push one of the balls towards the little finger with your thumb. The index finger, middle finger and ring finger should immediately start propelling the balls forward, while the little finger keeps pushing the outside ball towards the wrist. (You have to remember that we are once again working in an anti-clockwise direction with the right hand and in a clockwise direction with the left hand.)

Exercising with four balls demands great co-ordination between all the fingers of the hand. The better the movement of the fingers is co-ordinated, the better the exercise will succeed. This interaction is actually one of the goals which you achieve when you do this exercise. To work with four balls, you need a considerably higher degree of concentration and co-ordination than when you work with two or three balls. Working with two balls is mere child's play, in comparison.

At first, you'll notice that you feel just as clumsy as you felt the first time you started practising with two balls. Therefore, you'll realize immediately that you should not feel discouraged by your apparent clumsiness. You'll learn as you practise, and this applies to every exercise.

Obviously the exercise with four balls is also carried out with both hands, and in both directions. So you can start with the hand and the direction which you find easiest, and gradually make it more difficult for yourself, first by practising with the other hand in the easier direction, and then first with one hand and then with the other hand, in the direction which you find more difficult.

This exercise improves the circulation of the entire body, the operation of the central nervous system in general, and of the nerves in the arms and hands in particular; it strengthens the muscles and, because of the weight of the four balls, it has a more intense massaging effect on the reflex zones of the hands.

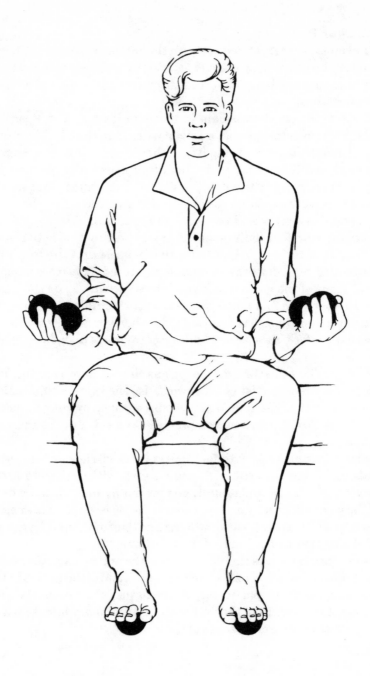

Exercises with the Feet
Place a rubber mat, or if you don't have a rubber mat, a blanket folded double, on the ground in front of you, and sit down in such a way that your feet just touch the ground when you relax your legs. Work with bare feet. Place a ball under each foot and roll it consecutively forwards, backwards and in circles in both directions. Start by going through the whole programme of movements with one foot at a time. It's only when you have acquired some dexterity with each foot individually, that you can start practising with both feet at the same time, moving them in the same direction. Then you can do the exercises moving the feet in opposite directions.
When you do this exercise with one ball with each foot, the size of the ball is not particularly important.
This exercise has the same effect on the feet and the legs as the exercises with the hands have on the arms and hands. They improve the sense of touch in the feet and heighten the sense of balance.
To make the exercise more difficult, you can work with two balls for each foot and with hands and feet at the same time.

Pushing Balls with the Feet
With your bare feet, try to roll a ball along the ground towards a goal you have chosen. You start using one foot at a time and then switch to both feet by hitting the ball alternately with the left and the right foot, rather like a footballer dribbles with the ball. You can try to push the ball alternately with the inside of the foot, the outside, the ball of the foot and the heel.
This is an excellent exercise for improving your dexterity. Make sure that you choose a suitable place. Some furniture does not take kindly to 'tapping the ball'; people living below might not like it either !

This exercise may also be carried out with two balls. In that case, each foot has its own ball to push forwards. It's not like a football match with long passes because your furniture – as well as the balls – might have difficulty surviving. Keep pushing the balls slightly forwards, alternately with the right and left foot. This is not only better for the furniture, as we already noted, but it also helps the exercise become more effective.
These exercises have a particularly good effect on rheumatic com-

plaints of the legs, problems with the circulation of the blood in the feet and legs (also, for example, for people who suffer from chronically cold feet) and for strengthening the muscles in the feet, ankles and calves.

Foot Baths with Ball Massage

A foot bath, particularly a foot bath in which the temperature is gradually increased, is even more effective if you place a ball in the water for each foot and move your feet to massage the soles of your feet with the balls. This has a twofold effect: because your feet are resting only on the balls, the soles of your feet have better contact with the water – and the circulation is more intensely stimulated by the soft massage of the soles. After use, rinse the balls thoroughly, dry them carefully, and rub them with oil. Don't use them in a foot bath if you have added any perfumed products or products based on salts. These substances are too harsh for the vulnerable surface of the balls.

Gripping Exercise

It is best to do this exercise with a large heavy ball, although of course you can use another type.

Start by practising with one ball in your more dexterous hand. Take the ball in your hand, so that the back of your hand is facing upwards and the palm is facing down. The hand is now holding onto the ball from above. If you open your hand, the ball will drop.

This is exactly what you should do.

Open the hand to drop the ball and then immediately clench your hand to hold it again. If you know that you won't succeed in this straightaway, and/or you have people living below you, it's a good idea to start by practising with a small squash ball. Make sure that there's a soft surface, and if possible, make the distance between the ball and the surface as small as possible.

For example, you could practise over your bed, or otherwise you can hold your other hand underneath. Once you have succeeded in doing this exercise without any difficulty with your more dexterous hand, switch to the other. Then you can start working with both hands at once. You can automatically catch the ball by folding your fingers around it. You can also try to catch it by holding the ball only with the palm of your hand.

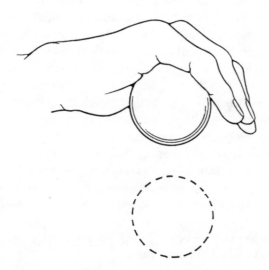

Refinement of the Basic Exercise
In the description of the basic exercises on pp. 57-59 we advised you to practise with the balls until you can rotate them in a flowing movement so that they don't collide, but constantly stay in contact with each other.
This is the easy way.
When a real master rotates the balls it looks different, but you can't practise this movement until you have used the easy movement for long enough so that you can do it in your sleep.
If you get this far, you can start on the real work. Allow the balls to roll through the palm of your hand, along the outside of the hands, *so that they do not touch each other*.
In order to achieve this, you obviously need to acquire greater dexterity, greater muscular strength in the hands and greater powers of concentration than those needed to do the easy variation of the basic exercise. The balls have to acquire more rotational force, and at the same time, the centrifugal force of their rotation should be used in such a way that they describe the largest possible circle on the surface of the hand, without falling.
The starting position for this exercise is more or less the same as that of the basic exercise (second step). One ball lies in the palm of the hand, the other rests on the bent ring finger and middle finger, and is balanced by the slightly raised index and little finger. Lift the ring finger and little finger slightly and push the upper ball to the thumb via the index finger. Keep the ball between the bent index finger and thumb and drop the other fingers slightly so that the other ball can roll round the outside to the ring finger via the little finger. At the same time, let go of the ball which is held by the thumb and the index finger, and push it down with the thumb, so that it rolls towards the heel of the hand via the heel of the thumb.
The way described here may seem complicated, but when you start to practise you'll soon find out how you can manage this best. Try to start by achieving a speed of ten complete rotations per minute and then try to gradually increase your speed to sixty rotations per minute.
In a competition held a few years ago in China, the champion achieved a speed of 200 rotations per minute.

Tai Chi and Chinese Health Balls
Chinese health balls can be beautifully integrated in Tai Chi exercises.
If you have any experience with Tai Chi or Qi Gong, you can imagine how an extra dimension can be added to these techniques with the use of Chinese health balls.
For those who have no experience in this field, we include a few practical tips.
The illustration on the next page shows a number of important ki points, which are relevant in these sorts of exercises.

The *starting position* is as follows:
Stand up straight with the feet parallel and slightly apart. Relax the knees so that they are slightly bent; relax the shoulders so that the arms hang loosely next to the hips. The head should be held straight on the neck, the spinal column is straight and relaxed and the whole body is in equilibrium. Focus your attention on the *Dantien* point, about an inch below the navel.
In each hand, hold two balls of the size which you find most comfortable to work with.
In this position, breathe in and out in a relaxed fashion. When you notice that you are breathing quietly, deeply and regularly, start directing your breath towards different places in your body. You do this by imagining as you breathe, that your breath is entering the body through that point or leaving the body through that point.
Start by breathing in at the Dantien point and breathing out through the Huiyin point (between the legs, just in front of the anus).
Now breathe in through the soles of the feet and breathe out via the lumber vertebrae.
Breathe in through the cervical vertebrae, breathe out via the outside of the hands (the Laogong point).
If you find it difficult to concentrate the breathing on a particular part of the body, practise this first in a relaxed way, before going on. Choose points for yourself which seem easy to you. You'll notice that after some practice, you'll be able to direct your breathing towards every part of your body.
Once you're able to use this method of projected breathing, carry out the exercises described here, and go on as shown below, with two balls in each hand.

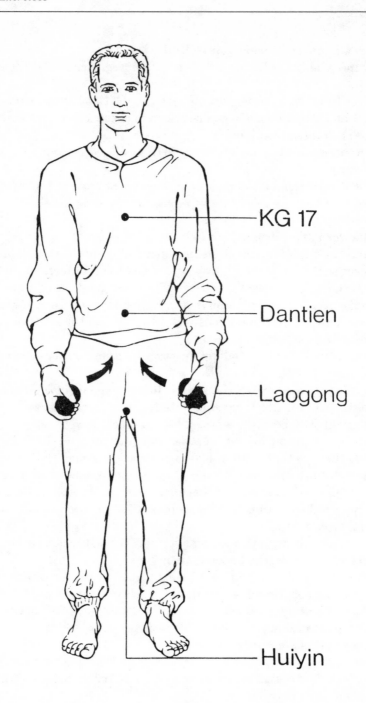

KG 17

Dantien

Laogong

Huiyin

One

Breathe in, and at the same time, raise the hands with the balls until you can roll the balls around. Raise the hands, rolling the balls, up to the KG 17 point, in the middle of the sternum. Now stop breathing. Hold your breath for a moment, drop your arms to the starting position, and at the same time, breathe out. Do this evenly and as smoothly as possible. Repeat the exercise three times.

Two

Next time, raise the hands again to the KG 17 point, and then move them from there to the side, until your arms are stretched out. From this position, slowly drop the arms back to the starting position while you breathe out. Repeat this exercise three times as well.

Three

From the starting position, breathe in and raise the hands with the balls to the KG 17 point, and spread the hands; at the same time, transfer the whole weight of the body onto the right leg. Now raise the left leg at the back, keeping your hands spread out (bird position). As you breathe out, lower the left leg, place the weight on both legs, and at the same time, drop the arms to the starting position.

Four

Now repeat exercise three with the weight on the left leg, while you raise the right leg to the back.

Five

Repeat exercises three and four alternately until you have done each exercise three times.

Six

Finally, stand quite relaxed in the starting position for a minute or two, and then breathe in at the Dantien point, and out through the Huiyin point, as in the beginning. All this should be carried out in a flowing movement, paying attention to every part of the exercise. At first, this will be by no means easy, particularly as you must rotate the balls at the same time. Again, it is important to take it easy. You can try to master the whole exercise first without using the balls; then repeat it with the balls in your hands, and finally repeat it again, rotating the balls. Do all this very slowly and take your time; it is not a matter of great achievement − it is a question of doing something for yourself, step by step.

All too often, in our behaviour and in our thoughts, we are concerned with external matters and achievements which have to be obvious to the outside world. Sometimes this means that we lose our perspective on things.

Working with Chinese health balls, and doing the exercises described here, will help you to achieve a balance within yourself. You will become more aware of your own body and the way in which it works. For example, very few people are aware that they are breathing, that there is such a thing as respiration. It is only when their breathing becomes less automatic, for example, in people suffering from asthma, that they become painfully conscious of this. However, an awareness of the way in which breathing and the muscles work can be felt in a much more pleasant way: by focusing the attention on it in a relaxed, agreeable way, exploring and feeling these sensations and training them with methods such as Tai Chi and Chinese health balls.

When you become more intensely aware of your own body, another form of consciousness also becomes clearer. Anyone who devotes attention to the balls and is prepared at the same time to see the exercises as a form of meditation, will find that it can give them an understanding of life.

The principle of the balls is a principle of co-operation. They only work as a unit when they are a pair, because it is only when there are two balls, that they can really be rolled around the hand. One ball pushes the other, and vice versa, and in this way they both help to keep the movement going. One ball cannot do this by itself, just as one person cannot achieve the same as two or more people can achieve together. One will set another into motion. One is all alone, a static unit, whether it is a ball or a person. You might object that a single ball could be rotated through the palm of the hand... but even then it is not the ball which achieves this through its own force. It's the hand which rotates the ball − just as it's the ball which massages the hand and stimulates life. It's the hand which warms the balls − and then the balls which heat up the hand and, via the hand, the body by means of their rotation and friction. Everything affects everything else, everything is interrelated, all things serve each other. Viewed in this way, the balls also serve in an exercise in philosophy...

Exercises for Dexterity

One
Practise with two balls in each hand, but do a different exercise in each hand. This will increase your powers of concentration.

Two
Hold one ball with five finger-tips. Press them together and then slowly relax. Repeat this a few times, with two hands as well. In this way, you'll strengthen the muscles of your hand. Then repeat the exercise with only your thumb or index finger. With your thumb, you stimulate the will; with your index finger, the power of thought.

Three
Place a ball on a soft surface underneath the palm of each hand and press the palms of the hand slowly but firmly downwards. Then relax. This is particularly effective for psychological problems and cramp.

Four
Take one ball between the palms of both hands and roll it between them by moving the hands (just as you would roll a meat ball). Do this with two balls at the same time and try to make the balls rotate around each other.

Five
Throw one ball up with your more dexterous hand and catch it. Then practise with the other hand, and then with two balls in each hand, and finally with two hands at the same time, first with one and then with two balls.

Six
Throw one ball up and catch it with the other hand. Change the hands. Then practise the same thing with two balls at the same time. Now place a ball in each hand and pass them to the other hand at the same time; repeat this with two balls in each hand. This is good co-ordination training.

Seven

Take a ball in your most dexterous hand, stretch your arm diagonally up and roll the ball towards your elbow along the inside of your arm. Catch it with the other hand. Also practise with the other hand. Let the ball roll on as far as possible; if you are very dexterous, you can finally roll it along the whole of your arm along the back of your shoulders, until it lands in the palm of the opposite hand !

Eight

In this exercise, the balls do not rotate around each other, but over each other. Spread your fingers and place one ball on the index finger and middle finger (A), and one on the ring finger and little finger (B). Slightly lift ball A, and press ball B against the bottom with the thumb, so that A is lifted further by B and B rolls underneath A. A rolls over B towards the thumb and is then pushed back underneath it towards the little finger, etc.

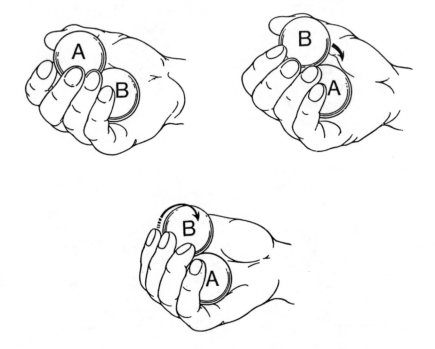

The exercise can also be done the other way round. In this case, ball B is lifted over ball A with the thumb and index finger, and ball A is pushed towards the thumb with the base of the little finger.
Do this exercise with both hands as well.

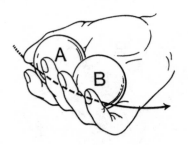

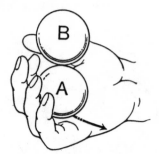

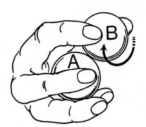

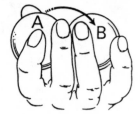

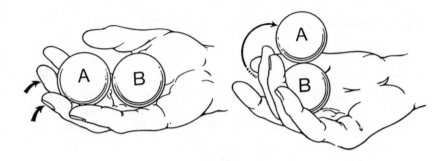

Nine

In this exercise the balls jump over each other. Ball A lies on the ring and middle fingers, which are spread out; ball B lies in the palm of the hand. Tilt the hand slightly back. Now make an upward movement with the wrist, and at the same time, push ball A with the fingers so that it is thrown over ball B, and lands on the heel of the thumb. Let it roll into the palm of the hand straightaway by tilting the hand slightly back again. A presses B onto the fingers. Repeat this a number of times. Practise this with each hand separately and if necessary with both hands at the same time. For this exercise it is also important to practise it above a soft surface.

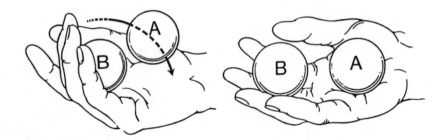

Meditation Exercises

One
Place the balls on the table in front of you on an attractive, softly coloured background. Sit down in front of the table in a relaxed position with your spinal column straight. Fix your gaze on the balls, and let go of your thoughts until you stop thinking altogether. Obviously you can do this meditation exercise in the lotus position, perhaps seated on the ground with the balls on a cushion or on a low table in front of you.

Two
Make a circle with the thumb and index finger of each hand and hold a ball with this. Keep the hands at the level of the nose, about one foot from the face, with the thumbs pointed towards each other (as though you are holding binoculars). Keep about two inches distance between the thumbs.
Now try to look between the balls with both eyes while keeping sight of both balls at the same time. This is a good concentration exercise in itself. Then let go of all your thoughts until they have disappeared, and try to meditate on the significance of the circle as a symbol of infinity and emptiness, and of the ball as a multi-dimensional infinity, in which each arbitrary point on the ball is at the same time the beginning and the end of an imaginary circle.

Musical Exercises

One
Start by holding one ball in each hand and moving them rhythmically until there is a sort of melody with chords. The longer you play with these, the more sounds you will discover. Also try it with two balls in each hand, and finally, with as many balls as you possess.

Two
Rotate the balls in your hand in the old familiar way, making sure that they occasionally tap each other. When you can regulate the rate at which they knock into each other, you can create a rhythm, and in a sense, a melody. With a few balls in each hand you can make the rhythm and melody more complex by doing something different with each hand. This is not impossible: musicians do it all the time. Try to concentrate on the sound to such an extent that you can hear individually what the left and the right hand are doing, but so that you also hear them both at the same time.
It's not only fascinating to play with sounds in this way; it's an exercise in concentration which will strengthen your perception and the co-ordination between the two halves of the brain.

Three
Wearing clothes that are comfortable, stand in the middle of the room. Make sure that there is enough space around you. Now carry out an improvised dance on the spot, with a ball in each hand. Let yourself be carried along by the sound of the balls and enjoy the rhythm, movement, action and feeling of relaxation. When you have finished dancing, sit down in a relaxed position for a while, rotating the balls softly in your hands.

Walking Exercises

One

When you are walking through the room, the garden, the park or wherever, take a ball in each hand and make it sound rhythmically at the rate of your footsteps, while your whole body also moves in this rhythm. Relax your muscles and allow them to follow their own movement.

Two

Take two balls in one hand or two balls in both hands. Then walk in the following rhythm; one step as you breathe in, rotating the balls three times - one step as you breathe out, again rotating the ball three times. Remember that you are walking slowly.

Three

Take two balls with you when you go for a walk and hold one ball against each ear in such a way that they block the ears. (Go for a walk in a quiet place). The gently fluctuating sounds stimulate the sense of hearing .

Four

As you are walking along, hold the balls in your closed hand. Focus your attention on the soft vibrations which the balls transmit to the fingers and the inside of the hands. These vibrations stimulate the sensitivity of the hand.

Five

Take a ball in each hand. Hold the hands with the palms facing down. Start walking along, and let go of the ball alternately with the left hand and the right hand, and then grasp hold of it immediately again. Do this in the exact rhythm of your walking pace.

Six

Repeat the last exercise, but make sure that you raise the right hand, let go of the ball and grasp it again, as you are putting your right leg forward, and then do the exercise with the left hand as you put your left leg forward. Slightly raise the hand which has let go of the ball, before moving it down again to grasp hold of the ball as it falls. This creates a rocking movement of the shoulders. Once you have mastered the whole exercise, you will notice that your whole body has assumed a rhythmically rocking movement. This is another very good concentration and co-ordination exercise.

Gymnastic Exercises

One
The starting position is on the hands and the knees with the hands
straight under the shoulders and the knees straight under the hips.
Hold a ball in each hand so you are leaning on the balls. Now push
your hands forwards a little so that the balls are acting like 'wheels',
and push them back again. Start with small movements forwards,
and roll further every time, making sure that your back remains
straight. If you suffer from back complaints it is better not to do this
exercise, or only do it in consultation with the doctor or physiotherapist.

Two
The same starting position as in the last exercise. Stretch out the left
arm from the shoulder straight in front of you so that you are suppor-
ted only by the right hand. Change over and repeat the exercise
several times.

Three
The same exercise as the last one, but this time as you stretch the left
hand forwards, stretch the right leg back, and vice versa. Repeat this
a number of times, at first a few times and later more often. These
exercises strengthen the muscles in the back.

Four
Take one ball in one hand and swing it round with a stretched arm.
Because of the centrifugal force, this strengthens the muscles of the
arm and loosens the joints. You can also do this exercise with two
hands at the same time. You can do all sorts of rhythmic exercises,
swinging your arms in this way. As your hands move down, let your
knees bend slightly.

Five
Stretch out on the ground and place a ball in the hollow of the front
of your neck. Try to press the ball down with your chin keeping the
back of the head on the ground. Do this movement very slowly,
moving the head back slowly. This is a good exercise for the vertebrae and the muscles of the neck.

Six

Stretch out on the ground with two balls next to each other placed under the neck. Press the neck down to the ground by pushing the chin down, keeping the back of the head on the ground all the time. The movement of the neck will press the two balls apart. This massages the neck muscles at the same time as stretching them. Repeat the exercise a few times.

Seven

Lie down on the ground on your back. Take one ball in each hand, with the palms of the hand turned face down. Slowly press down on the balls as hard as you can and then relax just as slowly. This exercise is good for the muscles of the shoulders and arms.

Eight

The starting position is the same as in exercise one, on the hands and knees. Press your bottom back until it is resting on the heels. From this position, place two balls perpendicularly under your nose then lower your head down to the ground as far as possible, with the nose pointing towards the knees. Push the balls forward with the back of the head. Raise your head, with the nose still pointing towards the knees, and lift your back as high as possible, like a cat when it is angry. Then push your bottom back again and rest. Then do the movement in reverse: with your back arched, move the head forwards past the balls, push the balls towards the knees with the forehead until your bottom touches your heels again.
Repeat the exercise once or twice. This exercise makes the whole spinal column supple.

Nine

Stretch out on the floor with a ball pressed between the feet. Slowly raise the ball with stretched legs, and then lower it again just as slowly. This is good for the muscles of the stomach and legs.

Ten

Lie down on the ground and place two balls on your stomach. Hold each ball with one hand, but in such a way that the balls can still move. As you breathe out, bring your stomach up as far as possible, and as you breathe in, pull the stomach in as far as possible. The balls will start rolling around when you do this; this movement, together with the vibration of the sound, massages the stomach and the organs underneath it. It is best to do this exercise with your stomach bared. Repeat several times.

Massage with Use of Health Balls

For this, you need the help of a partner, who does the massage. It is most pleasant to have this massage after a shower or a warm bath, when your skin and muscles are relaxed. Lie down on a comfortable, even surface, relax, and cover the parts of the body which are not being massaged, for example, with a bath towel. Make sure that the room is warm.

You can massage the whole body, but for special problems, it's also possible to treat only the problem area.

The general technique is as follows: the masseur takes one ball in each hand and rolls it over the skin of his partner. The balls can be rolled in a straight line, but you can also make rotating movements with the hands, so that the balls describe small, or even large circles or spirals.

You can work the neck and shoulder area in this way, with the person who is being massaged lying on his or her stomach in a relaxed position.

The whole back can be massaged in this way, first with small rotating movements from left to right, working from the spinal column down, and then in straight lines from top to bottom, and finally, in large circles, to the left and right of the spinal column, over the whole back.

Massage the legs (the front and the back) by rolling the balls from the ankles in a straight line to the groin, and then back to the ankles in small spiral movements. Repeat this a few times, until the whole surface of the leg has been massaged.

You can do the same with the arms.

On the front, you begin with the shoulder area with small circular movements, and then go on to the chest with larger movements. The soft part of the stomach is massaged with light circular movements. This can relieve all sorts of cramps and constrictions. Finally, roll the balls from the big toes upwards via the shoulders, down the arms to the little fingers, and then across the fingers and thumbs, along the inside of the arms, and down the sides of the body, back to the hollow in the sole of the foot via the other toes.

Part 5

Health Diary

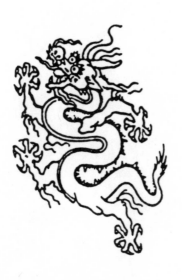

Your Own Memorandum
of Fun and Progress

In working with the health balls, you will certainly invent your own ways of playing and exercising with them. You will probably also note differences, even improvement, in the condition of your body and mind.

It might be a good idea to keep track of these improvements and, above all, to write down your own special discoveries and ways of working with the balls.

On the next pages you can make a start with your own exclusive exercisebook and health diary.

May pleasure be your steady companion!

Also published in this series

Eva Rudy Jansen

The Book of Hindu Imagery

The Gods and their Symbols

Hinduism is more than a religion; it is a way of life that has developed over approximately 5 millennia. Its rich and multicultured history, which has no equivalent among the great religions of the world, has made the structure of its mythical and philosophical principles into a highly differentiated maze, of which total knowledge is a practical impossibility.

This volume cannot offer a complete survey of the meaning of Hinduism, but Eva Rudy Jansen does provide an extensive compilation of important deities and their divine manifestations, so that modern students and anyone else who has an interest in Hinduism, can understand the significance of the Hindu pantheon.
To facilitate easy recognition, a survey of ritual gestures, postures, attires and attributes as well as an index are included.

Over 100 illustrations and several photographs make this book an important reference, both to the student of Hindu art and the interested amateur.

ISBN 90-74597-07-6 PBk.
ISBN 90-74597-10-6 cloth

Eva Rudy Jansen

Singing Bowls
A Practical Handbook of Instruction and Use

The Himalayan singing bowls, also known as Tibetan or Nepalese singing bowls, are a phenomenon which is fascinating more and more westerners with the singing sound of the metal bowls. By going to concerts, undergoing so-called 'soundmassages' and by experimenting themselves, people discover all sorts of possibilities and aspects of these special sounds.

This book explores these possibilities and aspects, tells something about the backgrounds, and provides practical information about the ways in which the bowls can be played, and how to choose a bowl for oneself.

It also contains an extra chapter describing three other ritual objects: tingshaws (small cymbals), dorje (thunderbolt) and bell.

ISBN 90-74597-01-7

The Book of Buddhas
Ritual Symbolism Used
on Buddhist Statuary and Ritual Objects

A brief introduction to Buddhism is followed by a lengthy survey in words and images of the most common figures, positions and symbols in Mahayana and Tantrayana Buddhism.

Each individual item is clearly illustrated and accompanied by a short description of its significance. Though it does not pretent to be complete, this book is nevertheless a valuable work of reference, providing anyone who is interested with an overall iconography of a world religion and its accompanying imagery, of which the philosophy and artistry have gradually also penetrated the west.

ISBN 90-74597-02-5

Also published in this series

Dirk Schellberg

Didgeridoo

Ritual Origins and Playing Techniques

The didgeridoo plays an important role in the creation myths of the original inhabitants of **Australia** – the sound of this wind instrument helped create the world and everything in the world. The deep, vibrating tones of this hollow pipe evoke a feeling of the powers of the earth, reaching more and more people outside of Australia.

The instrument itself is a miracle of simplicity. It consists of a pipe approximately as thick as a man's wrist. Authentic didgeridoos are made of eucalyptus wood naturally hollowed out by termites, and usually have a mouthpiece made of beeswax. The wealth of different sounds that an experienced player can conjure up with this apparently simple instrument can open up an entirely new world of experience for the listener. This book tells you more about the world of the didgeridoo – **its origins, the stories about the instrument and the players.** It not only deals with Australian musicians and bands, some of whom are gradually becoming popular in the West, but also discusses the experiences of Western therapists who have discovered new applications for the ancient sound. For anyone who is so fascinated by this sound and its possibilities that he or she would like to own a didgeridoo, the author includes practical instructions for building or purchasing a didgeridoo.

Above all, this book provides insight into the background and living conditions of the members of the ancient culture which produced the didgeridoo – the **Aborigines.**

ISBN 90-74597-13-0